How To Stop And Reduce Hair Loss

322 Great Tips To Prevent Hair Loss

ADAM COLTON

Published by BizMove
www.bizmove.com

Disclaimer

ISBN: 197844575X
ISBN- 978-1978445758

322 Great Tips To Prevent Hair Loss

You lose up to 100 hairs from your scalp every day. That's normal, and in most people, those hairs grow back. But many men -- and some women -- lose hair as they grow older. You can also lose your hair if you have certain diseases, such as thyroid problems, diabetes, or lupus. If you take certain medicines or have chemotherapy for cancer, you may also lose your hair. Other causes are stress, a low protein diet, a family history, or poor nutrition.

Treatment for hair loss depends on the cause. In some cases, treating the underlying cause will correct the problem. Other treatments include medicines and hair restoration.

Treating hair loss can be a simple activity if carried out in a responsible fashion. It is key to implement hair loss treatment knowledgeably in order to promote proper hair development and avoid causing damage to your scalp. The following suggestions pose a number of ideas about treating hair loss correctly. Implementing these pieces of advice will yield healthier, more beautiful hair.

1. If you are struggling with hair loss, it is a good idea to steer clear of tight hairstyles. The tight hairstyles

include buns, ponytails, and braids. If you keep your hair in a tight style, you will experience more hair loss. Try to keep your hair as loose as possible if it must be pulled up.

2. If you are a woman, birth control pills can result in hair loss. Look into some of the alternative methods of preventing pregnancy other than the pill. This will put you in a solid position to decrease the amount of hair that you lose during the course of your life.

3. It may just pay to wear a wig or toupee if you suffer from severe hair loss. Most hair loss medications are expensive and they do not always work the way people want them to. By getting a wig, you can pick the color, style and length of your hair.

4. Brushing your scalp will help stimulate hair growth. Vigorously brush dry hair. Scraping and rubbing your scalp will help to exfoliate the skin on your head. It will also help to increase the blood circulation in the scalp. The increased circulation brings nutrients to the hair, thus causing hair growth.

5. Calcium is a great supplement to receive if you're looking to strengthen your hair to prevent further loss. Calcium is essential in creating and

strengthening bones, nails, and even the substance hair is made out of, keratin. Make sure you're including some calcium-rich foods or a calcium supplement in your diet.

6. Rosemary and Sage are two herbs that are effective in treating hair loss. These natural herbs work by strengthening hair, which prevents it from falling out. To use this method properly, boil both the rosemary and sage in water. Then, strain the herbs and use it daily to see results.

7. Try medication. Hair loss medicines can slow hair thinning, as well as grow new hair and enlarge existing hairs. The medicines need to be taken continuously. If stopped, any new hair will be gradually lost, and in about six to twelve months your scalp will probably look about the same as before.

8. If you are losing your hair due to medications or aging, the best thing you can do is to simply accept that this is happening. You can be attractive without your hair. Move past the denial and accept that you are losing your hair, so that you can take steps to deal with the issue.

9. After shampooing your hair, rinse it with an apple cider vinegar and water mixture. This vinegar

mixture will simultaneously remove any extra debris left behind by your shampoo and nourish your follicles. Healthy follicles mean healthier hair, and your healthy follicles will have an easier time hanging onto your hair.

10.   Mixing castor oil and white iodine makes a potent solution that could help you to re-grow your hair. To make this concoction, simply add equal parts of each ingredient, mix them well, and then apply directly to the scalp (about a teaspoon's worth) and work to massage it in. Repeat this every night.

11.   Having toxins in your body can help speed up the hair loss process, so you should aim to drink at least 8 glasses of water daily to help strengthen your hair. Drinking this amount of water helps to purge your body of the toxins that can damage hair follicles. Once these toxins are gone, your hair can grow strong.

12.   A castor oil and almond oil mixture can help stop hair loss and make new hair grow in healthier. These natural ingredients work by making hair follicles stronger so that they will stay on your scalp. To properly use this method, just mix the two oils together and rub it into your scalp once a week.

13.   If you are emotionally affected by your hair loss, seek some counseling. You need a professional to help you cope with this problem which you have to live with. You do not want to let yourself be depressed over it because you can become preoccupied with it. This will lead to higher stress levels, which will only exacerbate the hair loss problem.

14.   Women tend to experience more hair loss due to dietary reasons than men do. Low iron diets and other nutrient deficiencies can cause hair loss in women. Make sure you are monitoring what nutrients you are getting out of your diet, and understand the concern to you as a woman.

15.   To keep from losing your hair, make sure you get enough iron in your diet. Iron deficiency not only causes anemia, it can cause hair loss. Fortunately, this is one of the simpler ways to lower your risk of hair loss. Take an iron supplement or eat more foods like clams, soybeans, pumpkin seeds and spinach.

16.   You should not use just any shampoo for your hair. You have to be careful which products you use on your hair. A good example is using a 3 in 1 shampoo, with a conditioner and body wash

included. This could damage your hair, which could lead to it falling out prematurely.

17.   Improving the blood circulation to the scalp is going to help you lessen the chances of hair loss. This can be accomplished by massaging your scalp with vegetable oil and then wrapping a warm towel around your hair for two or three hours a few times a week. It will increase the blood flow and prevent hair loss.

18.   When it comes to hair loss it is important to know the impact that genetics has on it. Hair loss can be hereditary. As such if someone in your family true suffered from hair loss, it is more likely you will too. Be informed and you'll have a better chance against whatever happens.

19.   If you're a vegetarian or anemic, a lack of iron in your diet may be the cause of your hair loss. You should check with your doctor and have your iron levels tested. If they're low, try consuming leafy vegetables, beans, or lean cuts of red meat to increase your iron level.

20.   The importance of vitamin C in preventing hair loss cannot be overstated. Vitamin C facilitates collagen production. Collagen is needed for healthy, living hair. If your consumption of vitamin C is

insufficient, remedy this by loading up on citrus fruits or popping a candy drop fortified with vitamin C.

21.   Living a stress free life will help you prevent hair loss. Stress can be a major cause of hair loss; if you don't know how to manage your stress, you may find yourself shedding hair down the drain. You need to learn how to handle stress.

22.   Taking an anti-depressant can sometimes have the side effect of hair loss. People routinely see themselves losing hair while on anti-depressants, as the ingredients in them may cause hair loss. You might want to speak with your physician to seeing if switching medications is an option. Perhaps taking a new medicine will halt the hair loss.

23.   Stress causes our body to release toxins. Stress is caused by many different things in our daily lives and through releasing these toxins, it directly causes change in our bodies. Hair loss is one of these changes, and while hair loss is also hereditary, stress is one of the combined factors that can affect hair loss.

24.   Apply gentle massage techniques on the scalp to help promote healthier roots and hair growth. Be careful not to pull or tug at your hair in the process

as this can pull out hair and cause breakage at the hair root. To ensure you don't pull your hair in the process, apply a conditioner before massaging to lubricate the scalp and rinse thoroughly when finished.

25.   There are two FDA-approved medications, Minoxidil and Finasteride, for treating inherited hair loss (androgenic alopecia).You can get Minoxidil (Rogaine) without a prescription. It is to sprayed or rubbed into the scalp twice daily. A prescription is needed for Finasteride (Propecia). Finasteride is not approved for women. It comes in pills to be taken once a day.

26.   Most people think that hereditary hair loss is about hair falling out. Actually, it's about more hair not growing back to replace shed hair. Genetic hair loss can be caused by gender (men suffer more than women) age and hormones (testosterone). Unfortunately, men do suffer the most.

27.   Vitamin B deficiency not only helps increase hair loss, but it can also cause premature graying of the hair. Without the proper amounts of vitamin B, your scalp becomes oily, full of dandruff, and begins to bald. Make sure you have enough Vitamin B by eating vegetables, grains, beans, and more.

28.   Your diet is worth serious consideration when you are dealing with hair loss. Foods that are high in carbohydrates are considered imbalanced foods which may result in unhealthy hair, even hair loss. Poultry and fish are low fat and high in proteins which aid in the health of your hair; don't forget fresh vegetables to infuse vitamins into your hair.

29.   A good portion of women may be surprised to learn that hormones can contribute to hair loss. Birth control can cause a hormonal imbalance, which could cause hair loss. A temporary hormone imbalance is created sometimes, even during hormone therapy. Checking your hormone levels and monitoring them over time is an important step in identifying the causes of excessive hair loss.

30.   To use lifestyle factors to prevent hair loss, avoid overusing certain unhealthy substances. Namely, eating too much salt, drinking too much alcohol and using too much of any tobacco product can all contribute to causing hair loss. Don't overindulge, and your chances of keeping a full, healthy head of hair will go up.

31.   One reason vegetarians and vegans lose their hair is because they eat too much soy and/or iodine. Soy can affect the thyroid, and thyroid imbalances are a cause of loss of hair.

32.   Combing and brushing your hair is going to help you reduce the risk of hair loss. If you use a wide tooth comb and a soft bristle brush, you are going to increase the blood flow to the scalp and it will also help to activate the cells of the scalp keeping it healthy and preventing hair loss.

33.   Avoid using anti-dandruff shampoos. Many people treat their scalps for dandruff when they do not actually have it. You will end up causing quite a bit of damage to your scalp if you treat it for the problem that it does not have. Dandruff is actually yellow flakes, not white powdery flakes.

34.   If you suddenly have unexplained hair loss, try to consider your life's stress level. Having a high-stress job or home environment may lead to abnormal hair loss. Thankfully, if you reduce your stress level, your hair should resume normal growth patterns.

35.   If you want to avoid damaging your hair, which could lead to hair loss, then don't use a brush on it when it's wet. It's best to just dry it with a soft towel, and let it dry naturally. Also, if you like to use a leave-in conditioner, keep the product away from the scalp.

36.   In order to help regrow hair that has been lost, you may want to consider purchasing an organic shampoo. Many times, hair loss is caused by the use of shampoos and other hair treatments, so it is important that you reverse this damage. Organic shampoos do that by cleansing your scalp and unclogging follicles so that hair can grow back.

37.   There is only one treatment for hair loss that has been shown to be effective and is FDA approved. That treatment is topical minoxidil and is the ingredient that is found in products like Rogaine. While studies aren't sure why it helps, they do know that it has been shown to strengthen hair growth.

38.   Ensuring that you diet has the appropriate amount of protein will help slow the rate of hair loss. Some good sources of protein include fish, poultry, nuts, beans and eggs. Eating these foods will help your hair produce keratin, which is its own protein. If your hair consistently receives keratin, it will increase in strength and resiliency, reducing your rate of hair loss.

39.   Vitamin E is a wonderful addition to your arsenal to combat the signs of hair loss. You can use this vitamin in oil form to moisturize your scalp and strengthen your hair. Additionally, you can take

this vitamin in pill form to reduce brittle hair that is prone to falling out.

40.   Lack of iron in your system can bring about hair loss. Iron is an essential nutrient for your hair and increasing your intake can slow the loss of hair. Green vegetables carry lots of iron and, though it may be hard for some to do, taking a couple of teaspoons full of black strap molasses can increase your iron intake. If the taste is not for you consider mixing it in your coffee.

41.   Think about starting out on a vitamin regimen in order to prevent further hair loss. Vitamins B, C, D, and E have all been known to help strengthen and fortify the chemicals in your body, as well as supporting your body's cellular growth. Starting a multi-vitamin regimen might just help you prevent hair loss.

42.   If you have long hair that you like to pull back in a ponytail, avoid the use of rubber bands or elastics that drag on the hair and pull it out. Instead, use soft fabric "scrunchies" where the elastic is covered, kept safely away from the hair shaft and won't tug on the hair.

43.   Be proactive about your hair loss. If you have longer hair and you notice it starting to fall out, get

a shorter haircut or consider shaving your head. This will make the hair loss less startling and prevent long loose strands from clogging your shower drain and ending up all over your home.

44.   Maybe being a little proactive with hair loss is the way to go here, if you know that you will inevitably lose your hair. You can reclaim a lot of power that baldness has over you, by simply making the choice to be bald instead of going bald. Shave your head and you can go bald on your terms, not nature's.

45.   If you have lost your hair and a wig isn't really your style, look into different types of hats and other head wear that you can use to make yourself feel better. It doesn't have to be a baseball cap or a Sinatra-like fedora. You can look into getting a turban or a scarf or some other type of head dress.

46.   A great way you can deal with hair loss is by speaking about it to someone. Some people out there really, truly love their hair and the thought of losing it "much less the reality of it" is incredibly devastating. Speak to someone about this and it may make you feel more accepting of it.

47.   One simple hair loss remedy that is often overlooked is a scalp massage. When taking a

shower or bathing, it is just a simple matter of massaging your scalp for a few minutes to stimulate circulation. This stimulates the hair follicles and helps wash away dirt and deposits that have accumulated throughout the day.

48.   Keep your hair trimmed. By doing this you are taking dead ends off of your hair and it can grow longer and healthier. Dead ends can prevent your hair from growing any more and can make your hair weak and brittle. This can lead to hair loss in the future.

49.   Do not dye your hair more than once every six to eight weeks. The more often that you dye your hair, the more damage you are going to do to both your hair and your scalp. If you dye it more often than this you are going to increase the risk of hair loss.

50.   Deep condition your hair weekly. You should be sure to condition your hair with a deep conditioner that contains protein. Do this at least once a week. A hot oil or olive oil treatment should also be used. This will help strengthen your hair and prevent hair loss in the future.

51.   Use aloe vera in your hair. For many years aloe vera has been used for hair health. You can mix it in

with your shampoo for the best results. You can also mix it with jojoba oil, castor oil or olive oil for good results. This will help soothe your hair and scalp.

52.   If you get stressed when you think about how much your hair might be thinning, consider just what arsenal of products you are putting into your hair. If you use products, such as gel or mousse, you need to wash them out at night. Essentially, hair loss can be caused by the clogging of pores by these products.

53.   If you are suffering from hair loss, you want to consider eating a healthier diet. Foods that are high in fat or sodium can actually cause hair loss. Foods that are high in vitamins and nutrients, like fruits and vegetables, can help promote healthy hair and regrow hair that has been lost.

54.   Try using Rogaine or another solution that contains minoxidil to help prevent hair loss. This is a topical solution that must be applied to the scalp twice a day, and it can be used by both men and women. Many people notice that after several months of use, their hair loss ceases. Some even experience a regrowth of hair.

55.   If you are a woman, birth control pills can result in hair loss. Look into some of the alternative methods of preventing pregnancy other than the pill. This will put you in a solid position to decrease the amount of hair that you lose during the course of your life.

56.   Liquid saw palmetto is efficient against hair loss. This product helps to keep DHT levels low, reducing hair loss by reducing this male hormone's effects. Juice the fruit and carefully apply the extracted juice to your scalp and hair.

57.   Aromatherapy is a great and effective way to help prevent and treat hair loss. The natural oils help to relax the scalp and promote stronger hair follicles. With this method, you will massage the oils into your scalp and leave it there for twenty minutes. After which, you thoroughly wash your hair.

58.   If you're thinking about purchasing a minoxidil product to assist in the re-growth of hair, aim for a generic brand. Generic brands will still give you the strong 5% minoxidil solution and the product will cost a lot less money. Never pay for the brand name. You're paying too much money for the same results.

59.   Take special precautions when you use hair treatments that could damage your clothing. Allow the product to dry before you allow your head to come in contact with anything.

60.   There are certain types of shampoos you can buy to aid in the prevention of hair loss, so these are a great option to look in to. Not only may these products help you to re-grow your hair, but they are also designed to be gentle on your scalp while cleansing your hair, so it's really a two-in-one product.

61.   If you want to prevent and stop hair loss, you could try to rub olive oil on your hair. The ingredients in olive oil help to make hair stronger and keep it from falling out. To use this method, you can simply apply a tablespoon of it into your scalp and massage it in. Wash it off after 30 minutes.

62.   There are many causes of eyebrow hair loss, such as too frequent eyebrow plucking and use of eyebrow pencils, as well as aging. If your doctor determines that your eyebrow thinning is caused by aging, you may use eyebrow cosmetics to hide the hair loss. If it's caused by certain medical conditions, you can use eyebrow Rogaine to diminish loss.

63.   See your doctor. Before resigning yourself to thinning hair, consult with your primary care physician. There are numerous conditions from hypothyroidism to vitamin deficiencies that could be the cause of your hair loss. If the hair loss is due to an underlying condition, treating the condition is often enough to restore hair growth.

64.   Relax. In cases of sudden or severe hair loss, stress is often the primary culprit. Take some time to relax and try not to worry as much. Relaxation techniques such as yoga, deep breathing exercises, and meditation can be very beneficial. Once your nerves have calmed, your hair can begin to recover.

65.   To control your risk of losing your hair, lower your risk of diabetes. Diabetes, like many diseases, is a fairly common non-genetic reason for hair loss. Cut the amount of sugar in your diet, watch your weight, and make sure that if you do have diabetes, you control it well. These actions will all help prevent diabetes-related hair loss.

66.   To keep from losing your hair, make sure you get enough iron in your diet. Iron deficiency not only causes anemia, it can cause hair loss. Fortunately, this is one of the simpler ways to lower your risk of hair loss. Take an iron supplement or

eat more foods like clams, soybeans, pumpkin seeds and spinach.

67.   To increase the health of your hair and possibly prevent hair loss, increase circulation to your scalp. You can do this by doing headstands, by giving yourself gentle scalp massages, by exercising, by breathing deeply or by improving your circulation in general. Better circulation to your scalp means more nutrients to your hair, and that means that you're more likely to avoid hair problems.

68.   Use satin or silk pillowcases. Many people believe by using this material to sleep on can prevent hair loss. Using cotton or flannel pillowcases can cause your hair to pull. A satin or silk pillowcase will let your hair slide around and won't pull on your hair, causing hair loss.

69.   Aim for around 60 minutes of exercise each day. Not only does working out help reduce stress, which has an impact on hair loss, but it also improves the circulation to your scalp. This helps your hair to grow and look beautiful. Exercise also improves your digestion, allowing your body to absorb nutritious foods that can improve your hair growth.

70.   Make sure to brush or comb every day. This is of course normal to do in regards to being well groomed, however, by brushing every day you will stimulate blood flow to the hair follicles. With the increased blood flow you can expect cells in your scalp to be more active and thereby increase hair growth.

71.   It might sound unbelievable, but if you avoid environments high in pollution, then you could actually be preventing hair loss. Pollution has been shown to cause damage to the hair because of the absorption of toxic substances into the body, and this increases the risk of hair loss.

72.   You want to avoid excessive alcohol usage if you want to prevent hair loss. It is a medical fact that damage to the liver can cause hair to fall out in both men and women. This does not mean that you cannot drink at all, just try to limit it as much as you can.

73.   For women who are worried about hair loss, avoid pulling your hair back tightly. The hair on the top and front of our heads is very sensitive and tend to be what are pulled the most tightly. This gradually brings the end of the hair follicle closer to the scalp, which makes it fall out easier.

74.   Use caution when you apply hair treatments to ensure you don't ruin any bed sheets and clothing. Make sure you give the product enough time to dry before letting your head touch anything.

75.   Maintain a balanced diet, including plenty of fresh fruits and vegetables. Keeping your whole body healthy will also keep your hair healthy, and healthier hair is likely to last longer. In addition, keeping your hair healthy will result in sleeker and shinier hair, improving your appearance.

76.   After shampooing your hair, rinse it with an apple cider vinegar and water mixture. This vinegar mixture will simultaneously remove any extra debris left behind by your shampoo and nourish your follicles. Healthy follicles mean healthier hair, and your healthy follicles will have an easier time hanging onto your hair.

77.   Making sure that you're eating foods rich in iron is a great way you can help strengthen your hair and prevent it from falling out. Think of eating foods like green leafy veggies, liver, dates, raisins and other dried fruits, and even whole grain cereals. These food sources are a great source of iron.

78.   If you are concerned about hair loss try lime seeds and black pepper. First, get equal amounts of

both lime seeds and black pepper then grind them up. Next, mix them with water. Then you can apply this mixture to your scalp. This should give you results you can see immediately.

79.   If you want your hair to stay beautiful, minimize exposure to toxins and pollutants. Toxic chemicals damage your immune system, decreasing your body's ability to function. Your system's struggle to stay healthy affects your hair, increasing the chance of hair loss. Outside pollutants can also affect your hair. Avoid breathing in paint fumes or exhaust and wear safety equipment whenever handling harsh chemicals.

80.   Keep your hair trimmed. By doing this you are taking dead ends off of your hair and it can grow longer and healthier. Dead ends can prevent your hair from growing any more and can make your hair weak and brittle. This can lead to hair loss in the future.

81.   Keep your hair clean. If you don't wash your hair your follicles can get clogged up with dirt and oil. This is what causes hair loss and can prevent you from growing hair back. You should be sure you don't over shampoo your hair because this can also cause hair loss.

82.   Aim for around 60 minutes of exercise each day. Not only does working out help reduce stress, which has an impact on hair loss, but it also improves the circulation to your scalp. This helps your hair to grow and look beautiful. Exercise also improves your digestion, allowing your body to absorb nutritious foods that can improve your hair growth.

83.   Rinse your hair with herbal tea. You can do this by steeping 2 bags of sage tea in about 8 ounces of water for 10 minutes. After you shampoo and pat dry your hair, apply the cooled sage tea mix to your hair. You will see instant results that will last.

84.   Take a high-quality multi-vitamin daily. This can help your body from becoming depleted of necessary vitamins. Your hair, like everything else in your body, depends on the proper levels of vitamins and minerals in order to grow. If your body is depleted, the results may be hair loss. Eating a wide variety of fruits and vegetables can also help.

85.   Hair loss can be experienced as early as your twenties and it can make you feel insecure or vulnerable. It will be important to make peace with this phase of your life. A shaved head has become a popular trend for men in the past few years.

86.   Avoid wearing your hair in styles like cornrows, braids or tight ponytails and do not use extensions while experiencing hair loss. All of these styles pull your hair tight, causing tension that can eventually lead to hairs breaking off or being pulled from the follicle, which is called traction alopecia.

87.   If you are experiencing hair loss you should be sure not to style your hair while it is wet or damp. Doing so breaks the hair and damages its elasticity by pulling it away from the root. Wait until your hair is dry to begin brushing it to prevent this type of damage.

88.   Fluctuating hormonal levels have also been linked to hair loss. Whether they are fluctuating due to a birth control pill, your time of the month, or menopause, changing hormonal levels have been shown to play a role in hair loss. If this is the case, it's important to not freak out because this hair loss is typically temporary.

89.   If you are a woman, birth control pills can result in hair loss. Look into some of the alternative methods of preventing pregnancy other than the pill. This will put you in a solid position to decrease the amount of hair that you lose during the course of your life.

90.   Make sure to avoid shampoo products that contain a lot of chemicals. These types of shampoos not only dry your hair out but lead to split ends and a damaged scalp. The next time you go to the drug store, purchase a shampoo that is made up of natural ingredients.

91.   Vitamin E is a wonderful addition to your arsenal to combat the signs of hair loss. You can use this vitamin in oil form to moisturize your scalp and strengthen your hair. Additionally, you can take this vitamin in pill form to reduce brittle hair that is prone to falling out.

92.   If you are pregnant and your hormones are causing you to lose hair, be sure to speak with your doctor or midwife before using any treatments. Many hair loss treatments are not safe for pregnant women to use and could cause serious side effects for both you and your baby.

93.   If you have a very hectic life, make sure that you find at least one hour during the day to exercise. Exercising helps to relieve stress and flushes out the toxins from your body. Aim to exercise at least three days a week to maintain a healthy head of hair.

94.   If you have long hair that you like to pull back in a ponytail, avoid the use of rubber bands or elastics

that drag on the hair and pull it out. Instead, use soft fabric "scrunchies" where the elastic is covered, kept safely away from the hair shaft and won't tug on the hair.

95.	In order to mitigate hair loss or see a substantial decrease in hair loss you need to eat a healthier diet. This means you should eat more fruits, vegetables, beans, and non-fatty meats like fish and poultry. Stay away from complex carbohydrates because they produce sugars that are harmful to your body's balance.

96.	Carbohydrate-rich food not only leads to weight gain in most people, it can also lead to hair loss in many, so try to cut back on the carbohydrates if you want to keep more of your hair. Carbohydrates get converted by the body into sugar, and higher blood sugar can result in quicker hair loss.

97.	Try to reduce your level of stress on your body if you want to slow down your hair loss. When your body is under stress, your body channels energy into repairing the body instead of growing hair. So the rate of your hair growth slows, causing your hair to thin. Try to treat your body with more care and do not exert yourself. You might see an improvement in your hair growth.

98.   To avoid undue alarm related to hair loss, be aware that birth control can affect your hair. Some women who have been taking birth control pills find that they experience hair loss when they stop taking the pills. This hair loss is temporary and is more inconvenient than a cause for real worry, as the body systems will automatically correct this type of hair loss.

99.   To avoid vitamin-related hair loss, don't take huge amounts of vitamin A. Vitamin A is good for you, but taken in extreme amounts, it can cause hair loss and can even be fatal to some people. Luckily, it's simple to avoid taking massive doses of vitamin A so this type of hair loss is easily corrected.

100.   To increase circulation, promote overall health and reduce hair loss, be sure to eat a healthful, balanced diet, drink lots of fresh pure water, get plenty of exercise and plenty of rest. Many times, people lose their hair due to stress and general lack of health. By taking care of your whole body, you will be giving yourself the best chance to keep a healthy head of hair.

101.   You can stimulate the scalp and avert hair loss with frequent gentle massage. Be sure to use the fingertips rather than using your fingernails since your fingernails may tear your hair. Use a small

amount of a natural organic oil such as carrot oil or olive oil to moisturize and nourish the scalp.

102.   Don't rub your hair. When you dry your hair you should be sure you don't do it too hard. Rubbing your hair too hard can make it come out easier. You should also avoid using a blow dryer. If you do use one, make sure you use it on low heat.

103.   You can make a pre-wash paste to use before you wash your hair to help prevent hair loss. You simple take henna with fenugreek, curd, egg and amala. Mix them into a paste form and apply it to the scalp. Allow it to sit for about five minutes prior to washing your hair.

104.   One tip to avoid the thinning and breakage of hair, is to avoid combing your hair with a fine-toothed comb when your hair is wet. Even though combing hair when it has just been washed is a tempting practice since hair de-tangles and straightens more easily when it is wet, this is a common cause of hair breakage and loss. The combing process applies immense stress on the hair's shaft, when it it wet and it weakens the roots of your hair.

105.   Stress has also been shown to have a link to hair loss. If you want to keep that full healthy head of

hair try to stay as stress free as possible. It has been shown that stress causes constriction and restriction of blood flow to the scalp, which causes hair follicles to die.

106.   A healthy diet is not only good for your body, but it is also good for your hair. Eating healthy foods ensures that your hair gets all of the vitamins and minerals that it needs. Often the body to shows poor health through the hair follicles and fingernails before it is shown in other parts of the body.

107.   If you color your hair, try not to color it too frequently. When you color your hair frequently, you are not allowing it the time it needs to recover from the last coloring session. You should aim for keeping a six to eight week gap between each time that you color it.

108.   While it might be hard, avoid styling products since you need to prevent losing more hair. These products often have chemicals that lead to your hair falling out.

109.   If you are a woman, birth control pills can result in hair loss. Look into some of the alternative methods of preventing pregnancy other than the pill. This will put you in a solid position to decrease

the amount of hair that you lose during the course of your life.

110.   Do not use any hair loss medications until you have discussed it with your doctor. While some over-the-counter treatments are safe, others may not be. Also, if you suffer from any medical conditions your doctor may tell you which hair loss treatments are safe for you to use and which are not.

111.   If you are taking a bath or shower, try to stick to lukewarm or cold water to wash your hair. Hot water can strip all the oils from your skin, which can yield the dryness and breakable hair. Only wash with warm water if you desire to have a healthy head of hair.

112.   If you are going to use hair styling products on your hair, make sure to take it all out of your hair at nighttime to prevent hair loss. Keeping these products in all night allow the chemicals to sink further into your scalp, which can make your hair fall out.

113.   As the week goes on, try to get as much fresh air as you can to help replenish your body with oxygen. If you stay indoors all the time, your hair will get

very damp and lose its texture. This will result in poor quality and can make your hair fragile.

114.   Make sure to wash your hair of any gels before you go to sleep. If you go to bed with gel in your hair, the pillow will often push the gel into the pores on your scalp. This prevents hair growth, and it also can damage already present hair follicles, making you lose hair more quickly.

115.   Many factors may result in hair loss, including certain illnesses and poor nutrition. If you have started losing hair and suspect it's not due to genetics, it may signify a thyroid or hormonal problem. Prolonged fevers are another culprit. Anemia and other vitamin deficiencies can cause both men and women to lose hair, as can low-calorie or low-protein diets. If you're not sure why you're losing your hair, it's a good idea to see if your doctor can diagnose an underlying cause.

116.   There are two FDA-approved medications, Minoxidil and Finasteride, for treating inherited hair loss (androgenic alopecia).You can get Minoxidil (Rogaine) without a prescription. It is to sprayed or rubbed into the scalp twice daily. A prescription is needed for Finasteride (Propecia). Finasteride is not approved for women. It comes in pills to be taken once a day.

117. You need to stimulate the circulation in your scalp every morning if you're hoping to re-grow hair. This doesn't have to be a full-on massage. You only need to run your fingertips across your scalp in a circular motion for at least three minutes. This will get the blood flowing and stimulate hair growth.

118. Before you start taking any herb that you've never taken before or using any hair loss product out there, it's always a good idea to speak to a doctor about it. You never know when you may have an adverse reaction from something you're taking, so it's always better to be safe rather than sorry.

119. To make your hair stronger and prevent breakage and loss, make sure you don't have a silicon deficiency. Silicon, a trace mineral, is necessary for healthy nails, skin and hair. The lack of silicon can make your hair brittle, which can cause thinning. Taking silicon can improve this problem within a few weeks. Food sources of silicon include apples, carrots, cereals, honey and almonds.

120. Keep an eye out for dandruff. Dandruff has a negative impact on both your hair and your skin. It is important to address the problem as soon as you

see it. There are a variety of home remedies, including using neem leaves and fenugreek seeks, that can help you get rid of dandruff and promote healthy hair growth.

121.   Consider switching products that you use for your hair if you have noticed your hair is starting to thin. If you are styling your hair with gel, mousse or similar products, it would be a good idea to wash these off your scalp and out of your hair before you lay down to rest for the night. Such products can clog follicles and cause hair loss.

122.   If you are struggling with hair loss you want to avoid combs and brushes with fine or metal bristles. This is because they can scratch and or irritate your scalp. As you are going through hair loss the last thing you and your thinning scalp need are irritations from a brush.

123.   It may just pay to wear a wig or toupee if you suffer from severe hair loss. Most hair loss medications are expensive and they do not always work the way people want them to. By getting a wig, you can pick the color, style and length of your hair.

124.   Consult your doctor to rule out a thyroid problem or anemia. Sometimes excessive hair loss

can be due to certain conditions, such as issues with your thyroid, lack of iron, or an excessive level of male hormones. Estrogen levels can rapidly drop after menopause causing elevated male hormones in a woman's body. If your doctor determines that these issues aren't the cause, then it is time to visit the dermatologist for a detailed scalp examination.

125.   If you are a man suffering from severe hair loss, you want to consider shaving your head. Not only will it be easier to take care of your hair this way, but you will prevent your hair from looking odd from hair loss. Also, it is the cheapest option available.

126.   Massage your scalp often to stimulate nerves and circulation. Scalp massages also help relieve stress, which is a major contributor to hair loss. There is no risk to trying this daily.

127.   Are you losing more and more hair each day? Are you fearing this hair loss will evolve into bald spots in the near future? One thing you can do to cut back on hair loss is the be more gentle with your hair when it is wet. Refrain from brushing or combing your hair roughly while it is wet. When wet hair roots are very weak and are prone to breakage.

128. Avoid the use of harsh shampoos if you are trying to save your hair. They can be incredibly drying and make the hair shaft rough and difficult to comb or brush. Use a shampoo formulated for babies or children for the gentlest cleansing and condition well after shampooing. If you use sticky styling products, brush your hair well before shampooing to remove as much of the product as possible and use a gentle clarifying shampoo occasionally to remove build-up.

129. One of the best ways to prevent hair loss is to prevent your hair from tangling, so it's best that you use a very soft pillow when you're sleeping. Make sure you purchase a pillow case that's smooth. Think satin or silk here. Also, never go to sleep with wet hair. This will cause massive tangling.

130. After shampooing your hair, rinse it with an apple cider vinegar and water mixture. This vinegar mixture will simultaneously remove any extra debris left behind by your shampoo and nourish your follicles. Healthy follicles mean healthier hair, and your healthy follicles will have an easier time hanging onto your hair.

131. What each individual needs for their nutrition depends on many factors including metabolism, age, diet, genetics, body size, and more. It is advised

that you seek advice from a medical professional as to what vitamin supplements you might need to take in order to help you prevent or stop hair loss.

132.   Women tend to experience more hair loss due to dietary reasons than men do. Low iron diets and other nutrient deficiencies can cause hair loss in women. Make sure you are monitoring what nutrients you are getting out of your diet, and understand the concern to you as a woman.

133.   Stop drinking caffeine. Caffeine can cause dehydration in your body which is the reason for hair loss. Although it's hard, you should try to replace any drinks containing caffeine with drinks like juice or milk. This will ensure your hair stays healthy and shiny and prevents more hair loss.

134.   To fight genetic male pattern baldness, take supplements. Male pattern baldness is thought by some to be caused by an interaction of testosterone and the natural oil in your hair -- basically, the interaction can reduce blood flow to your scalp. That decreases hair growth and keeps hair from being replaced as fast as it sheds. Supplements like zinc, saw palmetto, gingko biloba and pro-vitamin B5 are thought to prevent this kind of damage.

135.   You can make a pre-wash paste to use before you wash your hair to help prevent hair loss. You simple take henna with fenugreek, curd, egg and amala. Mix them into a paste form and apply it to the scalp. Allow it to sit for about five minutes prior to washing your hair.

136.   Eating spicy foods to increase circulation will work to prevent hair loss. Capsicum is found in cayenne pepper, and it can strengthen hair follicles, and stimulate hair growth. It also contains Vitamin A, a vitamin good for general health maintenance and a reduced risk of hair issues.

137.   The first tip to dealing with hair loss is learning as much about acceptance as possible. Hair loss happens to a great deal of people and by learning how to deal with it with confidence you will be able to look great no matter how much hair you have on your head.

138.   If you would like to avoid excessive hair loss, it's imperative that you keep stress levels under control. Stress is a big cause of hair loss, if you can't control it, you'll continue to have hair loss. Learn how to control your stress.

139.   Take Vitamin C supplements if you're suffering from hair loss. Vitamin C facilitates the flow of

blood to the scalp, while maintaining the capillaries that carry blood to hair follicles. More blood to the scalp means, hair will regrow even faster.

140.   One of the worst areas that you must avoid at all costs are locations with dry air. Regardless of the season, there are going to be places that are very parched, which can weaken your hair strands and make you prone to hair loss. Stay away from dry climates for the sake of your hair.

141.   It is vital to instill quality nutrients into your diet on a daily basis. With each of your meals during the day, make sure that you get a healthy dose of vegetables. Vegetables such as carrots will give your hair the minerals it needs to function properly and maintain strength.

142.   You want to consider laser hair restoration if you find your hair falling out. It is a safe way to get your hair back and it also makes new hair fuller and thicker. This treatment works by your dermatologist or doctor using a low level, infrared laser light on your scalp that encourages hair to grow.

143.   Henna is a traditional Indian herb that is useful for preventing hair loss. It works by repairing and sealing the hair shaft, which in turn, prevents it from breaking and falling out. Not only is Henna

effective, but it is inexpensive and can be easily found in health and beauty stores.

144.   Both high fat and low fat diets can contribute to hair loss. High fat diets increase the amount of testosterone in a male and low fat diets decrease the amount of testosterone. Testosterone levels that are not stable are what can increase the risk of hair loss, so you must balance the amount of fat in your diet.

145.   Using apple cider vinegar on your hair can prevent hair loss. Its natural ingredients help to keep hair healthy and in place. To use it properly, heat up the apple cider vinegar slightly. Then, pour a little on your hair and wrap it in a towel. Let it sit for an hour and then wash it out.

146.   Excessive stress can cause hair loss in men and women. Stress can be emotional, such as from the loss of a family member. Or, it can be physical, such as from an injury. If stress is a cause of hair loss, try to learn coping skills and try to cut down on work and lifestyle stress.

147.   Try a product containing minoxidil if you are suffering from hair loss. Shampoos or hair treatments with this drug may be effective against hair loss in certain people. You will have to keep using it to see if it helps your condition in the long-

term. The level of effectiveness can vary among different people, so monitor how you respond to it.

148.   Remember that excessive heat dries your hair and causes breakage. To prevent hair loss, avoid exposing your hair to excessive heat. Do not use overly hot water when washing your hair. Avoid blow drying or using heating devices such as curling irons. Also, protect your hair from the hot sun.

149.   To avoid thinning hair and hair loss, get enough antioxidants. Antioxidants are good for a lot of things, including improving the immune system and ridding the body of toxins, and when your body works better, it has more resources to devote to keeping every part of you healthy -- including your hair.

150.   One good piece of advice is to use olive oil and rosemary on your hair. Rosemary is especially important for healthy hair. It gives your hair volume, body and shine. The oil has also proven to exert an antioxidant effect on your scalp and hair follicles.

151.   Having healthier hair means that your hair is far less likely to fall out, and one way you can work to strengthen your hair is by limiting your salt intake. Try to avoid adding extra salt to the foods you eat

and always check the sodium content of food items if you're eating those ready-made meals and snacks.

152.   As your new hair loss will probably change your hair style and your overall look, it is important that you also look at new wardrobe choices. A nice polo and slacks looks great with most cropped hair cuts. Additionally, this entire look seems very put together but can be done in about 5 minutes.

153.   A great contributing factor to hair loss is hair style. Ponytails and other hair styles that cause the hair to be pressed too much can be a contributing factor to hair loss. The simple solution to this is just changing the style in which your hair is worn and you will avoid the loss of hair.

154.   A helpful strategy to diminish or avoid hair loss is to adopt better hair care habits. Avoid excessive dyeing and harsh chemical treatment to your hair. Refrain or limit the amount of heat applied to your hair through the use of blow dryers, curling irons, straighteners, etc. All of the above cause breakage of the hair shaft and can result in hair loss also.

155.   If you have recently been diagnosed with any type of illness, you have to work hard to take good care of yourself. If you choose to avoid medications that are needed, or avoid the doctor, there is a

chance that your body could ultimately lose the battle. It takes energy to grow hair, and if you are forcing your body to burn up all its energy merely to stay alive, you cannot expect to grow hair! This leads to hair loss.

156.   Do not use any hair loss medications until you have discussed it with your doctor. While some over-the-counter treatments are safe, others may not be. Also, if you suffer from any medical conditions your doctor may tell you which hair loss treatments are safe for you to use and which are not.

157.   If you have tried everything, you can help regrow hair from hair loss, you may want to consider surgery. There are a variety of different surgery options, and all of them are non-invasive. The most common is a microscopic follicular unit transplant, in which a doctor transplant follicular units to the bald area.

158.   The most essential foods that you can put in your body for your hair are fruits. Fruits contain a plethora of beneficial nutrients and complement any meal during the day or night. Eat fruit to obtain a high dose of vitamin C, which helps with collagen formation for your hair.

159. Aromatherapy is a great and effective way to help prevent and treat hair loss. The natural oils help to relax the scalp and promote stronger hair follicles. With this method, you will massage the oils into your scalp and leave it there for twenty minutes. After which, you thoroughly wash your hair.

160. Over-the-counter products won't work on all types of baldness, so don't put too much stock into one product to be a be-all end-all cure. You will need to do your research to avoid spending money on a product that won't produce noticeable results.

161. Calcium is a great supplement to receive if you're looking to strengthen your hair to prevent further loss. Calcium is essential in creating and strengthening bones, nails, and even the substance hair is made out of, keratin. Make sure you're including some calcium-rich foods or a calcium supplement in your diet.

162. If you want to prevent and stop hair loss, you could try to rub olive oil on your hair. The ingredients in olive oil help to make hair stronger and keep it from falling out. To use this method, you can simply apply a tablespoon of it into your scalp and massage it in. Wash it off after 30 minutes.

163. Honey is a natural ingredient that is effective in treating hair loss. When massaged into the scalp, it helps make hair follicles stronger, which reduces the chances of hair loss. You can use a tablespoon directly onto your scalp or you can mix it in with your shampoo or conditioner.

164. DHT is the byproduct of testosterone breakdown and is the major factor in hair loss. This actually means that hair loss is due mostly to a hormonal imbalance. Many studies have shown that this is true, including one test among Japanese men who ate westernized diets. Improve your diet today.

165. One of the best ways to prevent hair loss is to prevent your hair from tangling, so it's best that you use a very soft pillow when you're sleeping. Make sure you purchase a pillow case that's smooth. Think satin or silk here. Also, never go to sleep with wet hair. This will cause massive tangling.

166. You must take action to get rid of the stress you are under. Hair loss has been directly linked to stress. The more stressed you are, the better chance you have for losing your hair. It can also make it harder to halt hair loss that has already begun, as well as making treatments ineffective.

167.   Try a product containing minoxidil if you are suffering from hair loss. Shampoos or hair treatments with this drug may be effective against hair loss in certain people. You will have to keep using it to see if it helps your condition in the long-term. The level of effectiveness can vary among different people, so monitor how you respond to it.

168.   To prevent hair loss, massage your scalp. Massaging the roots of your hair for five minutes every day increases the circulation to your hair follicles. This ensures a healthy supply of blood, and healthy follicles produce healthy hair. You can massage your scalp using an electric massager, but it is not necessary. Often you will find your fingers can do a perfectly good job.

169.   To increase the health of your hair and possibly prevent hair loss, increase circulation to your scalp. You can do this by doing headstands, by giving yourself gentle scalp massages, by exercising, by breathing deeply or by improving your circulation in general. Better circulation to your scalp means more nutrients to your hair, and that means that you're more likely to avoid hair problems.

170.   When you style your hair, don't pull it back tightly or brush it excessively. Gently coax it into place and leave it a little loose to avoid breakage and

hair loss. Be sure to use gentle hair styling devices that are free of sharp edges, and never use plain rubber bands to hold your hair in place.

171.   Make sure you drink enough water daily. Water can help get rid of toxins in your body that could be contributing to hair loss. You should drink at least 14 glasses of water that is filtered and without chlorine and lead. Water can help prevent hair loss in the future.

172.   When it comes to hair loss it is important to know the impact that genetics has on it. Hair loss can be hereditary. As such if someone in your family true suffered from hair loss, it is more likely you will too. Be informed and you'll have a better chance against whatever happens.

173.   Try using Rogaine or another solution that contains minoxidil to help prevent hair loss. This is a topical solution that must be applied to the scalp twice a day, and it can be used by both men and women. Many people notice that after several months of use, their hair loss ceases. Some even experience a regrowth of hair.

174.   Contrary to popular belief, it is important that you wash your hair daily. By not washing your hair everyday, you are allowing sebum to build on your

scalp, which in turn, causes hair loss. If you are concerned about washing your hair daily, you could try using a gentle shampoo or conditioner.

175.   A great way to help stop hair loss is to massage your scalp. Scalp massages will increase blood flow and circulation which will prevent hair loss. Make sure that for five to ten minutes, you massage your entire scalp. This is also a good way to reduce your stress, which can lead to hair loss too.

176.   Infra-red and UV light treatments are new hair loss treatments. These treatments do not work for every body. The only consistent results have been shown by those with very mild hair loss and those who are just beginning to lose their hair. This may be something that could work for your.

177.   As the week goes on, try to get as much fresh air as you can to help replenish your body with oxygen. If you stay indoors all the time, your hair will get very damp and lose its texture. This will result in poor quality and can make your hair fragile.

178.   Calcium is a great supplement to receive if you're looking to strengthen your hair to prevent further loss. Calcium is essential in creating and strengthening bones, nails, and even the substance hair is made out of, keratin. Make sure you're

including some calcium-rich foods or a calcium supplement in your diet.

179.   Natural herbal supplements to grow back your hair are the way to go for people who want to avoid the side effects associated with traditional medications. Some supplements will obviously work better than others, so you will need to test each one out individually to see what works best for you.

180.   Using apple cider vinegar on your hair can prevent hair loss. Its natural ingredients help to keep hair healthy and in place. To use it properly, heat up the apple cider vinegar slightly. Then, pour a little on your hair and wrap it in a towel. Let it sit for an hour and then wash it out.

181.   If you start losing your hair, stop any chemical treatments on your hair. This includes coloring and perms. The chemicals used in these treatments will dry out your hair, which results in your hair falling out faster. While coloring will give you a temporary effect of thicker hair, it is an illusion that will not last.

182.   If you are about to embark on a round of chemotherapy, losing your hair may be an undesired side effect. If you are concerned about hair loss, talk to your doctor or oncologist about the cocktail of

drugs you will be taking. Request that he looks into a mixture of chemotherapy drugs that will offer tumor shrinkage with fewer chances of hair loss. Preventing hair loss can really boost a cancer patient's outlook!

183.   Hair shafts breaking can be caused by many things, and this triggers thin hair, which ultimately results in weak structure and hair loss. Chlorine, chemicals, sun, and excessive styling are just some of the things that can cause this type of problem. Make sure you are taking proper care of your hair so this does not happen.

184.   When you style your hair, don't pull it back tightly or brush it excessively. Gently coax it into place and leave it a little loose to avoid breakage and hair loss. Be sure to use gentle hair styling devices that are free of sharp edges, and never use plain rubber bands to hold your hair in place.

185.   Eat protein. Protein adds an excellent boost to your diet and helps the way your hair will look and grow. It strengthens hair and prevents it from falling out. Eat things like fish, meat and nuts for protein. You can also use a protein supplement in your drinks every day.

186. Take vitamins for your skin and hair health. While these are not effective immediately and will take a couple of months to work, they are well worth the wait. Take vitamins or supplements that have Vitamin B in them for the best hair health. Be patient for the results.

187. While hair loss is mainly associated strictly with men it is possible to have this in some female cases as well. Normally it starts much later in women than in men and it can often be more difficult to deal with for a woman. There are many treatments to help a woman with this.

188. See your doctor if you're losing your hair. Thyroid problems are one of the number one causes of diffuse hair loss. Your doctor can perform a blood test to check for this. In the event that you need it, he or she can also write a prescription for medication that will help. Once your thyroid is fixed, your hair loss will stop.

189. Try using Rogaine or another solution that contains minoxidil to help prevent hair loss. This is a topical solution that must be applied to the scalp twice a day, and it can be used by both men and women. Many people notice that after several months of use, their hair loss ceases. Some even experience a regrowth of hair.

190.   Make sure to brush or comb every day. This is of course normal to do in regards to being well groomed, however, by brushing every day you will stimulate blood flow to the hair follicles. With the increased blood flow you can expect cells in your scalp to be more active and thereby increase hair growth.

191.   The most essential foods that you can put in your body for your hair are fruits. Fruits contain a plethora of beneficial nutrients and complement any meal during the day or night. Eat fruit to obtain a high dose of vitamin C, which helps with collagen formation for your hair.

192.   Drugs will work to weaken the roots of your hair at the follicle, so you should avoid drugs and alcohol if you're hoping to strengthen your hair and scalp and to prevent any further hair loss. Make this sacrifice and your hair will become much stronger in the long run.

193.   Apply gentle massage techniques on the scalp to help promote healthier roots and hair growth. Be careful not to pull or tug at your hair in the process as this can pull out hair and cause breakage at the hair root. To ensure you don't pull your hair in the process, apply a conditioner before massaging to

lubricate the scalp and rinse thoroughly when finished.

194.   Hair and nails are made of keratin, which derives from protein. Make sure that you have enough protein in your diet. The best way to get a lot of protein in your diet is from meats and poultry, but if you are a vegetarian you should consider taking a supplement.

195.   Be proactive about your hair loss. If you have longer hair and you notice it starting to fall out, get a shorter haircut or consider shaving your head. This will make the hair loss less startling and prevent long loose strands from clogging your shower drain and ending up all over your home.

196.   After shampooing your hair, rinse it with an apple cider vinegar and water mixture. This vinegar mixture will simultaneously remove any extra debris left behind by your shampoo and nourish your follicles. Healthy follicles mean healthier hair, and your healthy follicles will have an easier time hanging onto your hair.

197.   Look for reasons that may have contributed to your hair loss. A medication you have been taking or a stressful event could cause a loss of hair. If you

can think of a specific reason for your hair loss, you might be able to take steps to fix the problem.

198.   Be sure you are getting enough protein in your diet. If your follicles aren't getting enough protein, they move into a resting phase in which no new hair growth takes place. If new hair isn't growing in, the old hair will fall out. Eating a balanced diet with enough protein can prevent this cycle.

199.   If you are emotionally affected by your hair loss, seek some counseling. You need a professional to help you cope with this problem which you have to live with. You do not want to let yourself be depressed over it because you can become preoccupied with it. This will lead to higher stress levels, which will only exacerbate the hair loss problem.

200.   Try using coconut milk or aloe vera. You can use either one for this. First you massage coconut milk or aloe vera gel gently into your hair. You should leave this in your hair for 30 minutes. Next, you should rinse it off with warm water. Repeat three times a week for the best results.

201.   See your doctor. Before resigning yourself to thinning hair, consult with your primary care physician. There are numerous conditions from

hypothyroidism to vitamin deficiencies that could be the cause of your hair loss. If the hair loss is due to an underlying condition, treating the condition is often enough to restore hair growth.

202.   For healthier hair and less hair loss, consider using shampoos and hair products specifically designed to prevent hair loss. There are many hair products on the market containing ingredients that scientific research indicates may help prevent hair loss, like amino acids, B vitamins and zinc. These products can help some people see reduced hair loss and increased hair growth.

203.   A grooming tip which can prevent the thinning and breakage of hair is to avoid a hair style that pulls the hair tight. Many people, especially women, choose a hair style where the hair is pulled back tightly and is held there with a fastening device such as an elastic band or barrette. Styling your hair in this manner causes friction between the strands of hair and results in the breakage and thinning of hair.

204.   Calcium is going to play a big role in whether you suffer from hair loss. Low levels of calcium in your diet could lead to weak hair follicles and hair roots which will cause your hair to begin to fall out. Increase the amount of calcium in your diet to prevent the hair from falling out.

205.   When it comes to hair loss it is important to know the impact that genetics has on it. Hair loss can be hereditary. As such if someone in your family true suffered from hair loss, it is more likely you will too. Be informed and you'll have a better chance against whatever happens.

206.   To help stave off hair loss be cautious with the types of chemicals and treatments you put on it. Many dyes have chemicals in them that are not good for your hair. Trust your hair to a licensed beautician, and you may be able to prevent some hair loss before it starts.

207.   If you're a vegetarian or anemic, a lack of iron in your diet may be the cause of your hair loss. You should check with your doctor and have your iron levels tested. If they're low, try consuming leafy vegetables, beans, or lean cuts of red meat to increase your iron level.

208.   Not all hair products are healthy to your hair. If you choose wisely, and are aware of what products cause damage, you will be okay. Certain products can inhibit hair growth. Use only products that have been researched and proven harmless to humans.

209.   If you are on the swim team in high school or college, or you just like to use the pool a lot, refrain from staying underwater too long. Soaking your hair in water for a long time can lead to dryness and hair loss. Wearing a swimming cap can really help. Use a quality conditioner to help to protect your hair.

210.   Find a medicated shampoo or hair treatment that works for you. There are several top products on the market. That doesn't mean, however, that these products are going to work for you. It may take a specialist consultation or a bit of research or experimentation, but you should find something that gives you results more so than everyone else. Everyone is different.

211.   A ponytail is a great way to pull hair back and keep it neat, but be careful to move the position of the your ponytail on a daily basis. Hair that is constantly stressed in the same spot by ponytail holders, barrettes and headbands, can be easily weakened and break or fall out.

212.   In order to mitigate hair loss or see a substantial decrease in hair loss you need to eat a healthier diet. This means you should eat more fruits, vegetables, beans, and non-fatty meats like fish and poultry. Stay away from complex carbohydrates because

they produce sugars that are harmful to your body's balance.

213.   If you're applying monixidil to your hair in order to get it to grow, make sure you do this very early in the morning if you're going to work. It takes a solid three hours for this product to dry, and it can make your hair look very sticky and unappealing. It's only a cosmetic issue, but you may not want to run around with nasty-looking hair.

214.   Stress is disputed depending on who you talk to, but many people agree that excess stress levels can lead to hair loss. At the very least, having increased levels of stress will work to counteract any products you're taking to assist in hair growth. Make sure you work on your stress if you want to grow your hair back.

215.   Alopecia areata, caused when hair follicles are attacked by the immune system, can be treated with corticosteroids. Corticosteroids may be injected into the scalp every 4 to 6 weeks and are best for patchy hair loss. Corticosteroid creams or ointments may be used with injected steroids or other medicines such as minoxidil. Oral corticosteroids are rarely used because of side effects.

216.   Vitamin B deficiency not only helps increase hair loss, but it can also cause premature graying of the hair. Without the proper amounts of vitamin B, your scalp becomes oily, full of dandruff, and begins to bald. Make sure you have enough Vitamin B by eating vegetables, grains, beans, and more.

217.   To fight genetic male pattern baldness, take supplements. Male pattern baldness is thought by some to be caused by an interaction of testosterone and the natural oil in your hair -- basically, the interaction can reduce blood flow to your scalp. That decreases hair growth and keeps hair from being replaced as fast as it sheds. Supplements like zinc, saw palmetto, gingko biloba and pro-vitamin B5 are thought to prevent this kind of damage.

218.   A grooming tip which can prevent the thinning and breakage of hair is to avoid a hair style that pulls the hair tight. Many people, especially women, choose a hair style where the hair is pulled back tightly and is held there with a fastening device such as an elastic band or barrette. Styling your hair in this manner causes friction between the strands of hair and results in the breakage and thinning of hair.

219.   Maintaining your overall health is going to help you reduce the chances of hair loss. If you take care of your body, you are also taking care of your scalp.

Getting the right amount of sleep and eating a healthy diet is going to reduce the chances of suffering from hair loss.

220.   Protect your scalp from the sun. Sunburn is going to cause a great deal of damage to the follicles. Be sure to wear a loose fitting hat when you are out in the sun to prevent the burn and avoid damaging the follicles. If you have a bald spot, be sure to apply sunscreen to it in addition to wearing a hat.

221.   Stress has also been shown to have a link to hair loss. If you want to keep that full healthy head of hair try to stay as stress free as possible. It has been shown that stress causes constriction and restriction of blood flow to the scalp, which causes hair follicles to die.

222.   If you are suffering from hair loss, you want to consider eating a healthier diet. Foods that are high in fat or sodium can actually cause hair loss. Foods that are high in vitamins and nutrients, like fruits and vegetables, can help promote healthy hair and regrow hair that has been lost.

223.   Some hair styles can cause hair loss. Pulling the hair tightly, or pulling it back in a hair band for quite a period of time, should be avoided. Although

hair products are much better than they used to be, they can still damage you hair. If you wear your hair in a tight ponytail, it can damage both the hair shaft and the hair follicles.

224.   In order to avoid hair loss women should avoid hairstyles that pull the hair tight. Braiding and weaving the hair can cause pus filled bumps to form on the scalp. These bumps then form scars and lead to permanent hair loss.

225.   Although you may use a lot of hair spray and mousse products, you should avoid these if you're losing your hair. They can simply be too harsh on your scalp and can ultimately damage your hair follicles and cause your hair to fall out. Until you can strengthen your hair, avoid the harsh products.

226.   Take Vitamin E supplements if you are suffering from hair loss. Vitamin E promotes healthy blood circulation, which, in turn, promotes healthy hair growth. It will also have the added benefit of keeping your skin healthy and youthful looking.

227.   Both high fat and low fat diets can contribute to hair loss. High fat diets increase the amount of testosterone in a male and low fat diets decrease the amount of testosterone. Testosterone levels that are

not stable are what can increase the risk of hair loss, so you must balance the amount of fat in your diet.

228.   DHT is the byproduct of testosterone breakdown and is the major factor in hair loss. This actually means that hair loss is due mostly to a hormonal imbalance. Many studies have shown that this is true, including one test among Japanese men who ate westernized diets. Improve your diet today.

229.   The herb basil has strong properties which could help you to prevent further hair loss or even aid in the re-growth of your hair. Crush about 20 fresh basil leaves and then put them into a glass or two of warm water. Allow this mixture to steep and cool. Then put it into a spray bottle and wet your hair with it at least twice a day.

230.   In order to help prevent hair loss, make sure you are getting enough protein in your diet. To keep your hair as healthy as possible, try to eat plenty of protein-rich foods as often as you can. Some good sources of foods rich in protein include eggs, seafood, bean sprouts, almonds, and fish.

231.   Illness, stress, anemia, weight change, and more can cause hair loss, temporarily. This temporary hair loss often starts 3 months after an event ends, and usually lasts about 3 months in total. Know these

things and keep them in mind if you experience hair loss.

232.   Try to keep yourself from being stressed out. Having stress can lead to hair loss and early gray hair. You can avoid the stress by using methods like meditation or yoga. This will help keep stress levels down and help you with maintaining your hair and not losing any more.

233.   To prevent hair loss, massage your scalp. Massaging the roots of your hair for five minutes every day increases the circulation to your hair follicles. This ensures a healthy supply of blood, and healthy follicles produce healthy hair. You can massage your scalp using an electric massager, but it is not necessary. Often you will find your fingers can do a perfectly good job.

234.   To use lifestyle factors to prevent hair loss, avoid overusing certain unhealthy substances. Namely, eating too much salt, drinking too much alcohol and using too much of any tobacco product can all contribute to causing hair loss. Don't overindulge, and your chances of keeping a full, healthy head of hair will go up.

235.   To prevent hair damage and thus lower the potential for hair loss, get more vitamin B. Vitamin

B and B complex vitamins in general strengthen hair follicles, which reduces the risk of hair damage, thinning and loss. Vitamin B may also help boost hair growth, too. It is found in a variety of foods, including spinach, red bell peppers and garlic.

236.   Be sure to use nourishing, natural shampoos if you are worried about hair loss. Be sure the shampoo you choose does not contain drying ingredients such as alcohol. If your hair and scalp are very dry, simply wash your hair gently with a natural, organic conditioner and skip the shampoo altogether.

237.   One tip to avoid the thinning and breakage of hair, is to avoid combing your hair with a fine-toothed comb when your hair is wet. Even though combing hair when it has just been washed is a tempting practice since hair de-tangles and straightens more easily when it is wet, this is a common cause of hair breakage and loss. The combing process applies immense stress on the hair's shaft, when it it wet and it weakens the roots of your hair.

238.   One of the best ways to limit hair loss is to reduce the amount of stress in your life. If you are at a job that puts you under a lot of pressure, make sure to practice stress relieving exercises during the

day. This will make you feel better and help hair loss.

239.   If you color your hair, try not to color it too frequently. When you color your hair frequently, you are not allowing it the time it needs to recover from the last coloring session. You should aim for keeping a six to eight week gap between each time that you color it.

240.   Vitamin E is a wonderful addition to your arsenal to combat the signs of hair loss. You can use this vitamin in oil form to moisturize your scalp and strengthen your hair. Additionally, you can take this vitamin in pill form to reduce brittle hair that is prone to falling out.

241.   Castor oil can be a natural safeguard in your hair loss defense. Mixing a teaspoon of castor oil with an herbal shampoo can increase volume and density in the hair and create a more manageable hair shaft. Stay away from shampoos with assorted chemicals, as this will negate the usefulness of the oil. You can see a decrease in your hair loss after a few applications.

242.   In order to prevent your hair from falling out, you want to consider avoiding hair relaxers. The chemicals in these products are known to make hair

fragile and fall out. Also, avoid using rollers in your hair. They grab onto hair too tightly and could cause it to fall out.

243.   Drugs will work to weaken the roots of your hair at the follicle, so you should avoid drugs and alcohol if you're hoping to strengthen your hair and scalp and to prevent any further hair loss. Make this sacrifice and your hair will become much stronger in the long run.

244.   Be ready for a lifelong application process if you opt for Rogaine or any Rogaine-like medicine. As soon as you stop using these products, your hair will again weaken and begin to fall out. Products like these counteract the genetic causes of hair loss, but only as long as you're using them.

245.   Exercise is essential not only for a healthy overall lifestyle, but also to help re-grow your hair. Because your scalp needs ample oxygen and blood flow in order to grow strong, healthy hair, exercising more will boost this and allow for your scalp to produce solid hair follicles that ultimately lead to stronger hair.

246.   Avoid hair dryers and flat irons if you want to prevent hair loss. The heat from these products can dry out your hair and make it fall out. If you have to

use them, be sure that you have them both on a low setting.

247.   Try to keep yourself from being stressed out. Having stress can lead to hair loss and early gray hair. You can avoid the stress by using methods like meditation or yoga. This will help keep stress levels down and help you with maintaining your hair and not losing any more.

248.   To increase circulation, promote overall health and reduce hair loss, be sure to eat a healthful, balanced diet, drink lots of fresh pure water, get plenty of exercise and plenty of rest. Many times, people lose their hair due to stress and general lack of health. By taking care of your whole body, you will be giving yourself the best chance to keep a healthy head of hair.

249.   When you style your hair, don't pull it back tightly or brush it excessively. Gently coax it into place and leave it a little loose to avoid breakage and hair loss. Be sure to use gentle hair styling devices that are free of sharp edges, and never use plain rubber bands to hold your hair in place.

250.   Treat your hair gently to avoid hair loss. After gently washing and conditioning your hair, wrap it gently in a warm towel and allow excess water to

blot off. Once your hair is just slightly damp, comb it out gently with a wide toothed comb and allow it to air dry naturally rather than using a hot blow dryer.

251. You can stimulate the scalp and avert hair loss with frequent gentle massage. Be sure to use the fingertips rather than using your fingernails since your fingernails may tear your hair. Use a small amount of a natural organic oil such as carrot oil or olive oil to moisturize and nourish the scalp.

252. To prevent hair loss through nutrient deficiency, make sure to get enough of the amino acid lysine. Lysine deficiency has been linked to hair loss problems, while increased lysine intake has been linked to increased hair growth rate and decreased shedding of hair. Lysine is available in supplements, but is also found in foods, such as yogurt, cheese, beets and mangos.

253. Take vitamins daily. Since hair loss can be caused by a diet that lacks nutrients, you should be sure to get a multivitamin daily. Take one that easily absorbs into the adult body. This will help replenish necessary vitamins and nutrients in your diet that can be contributing to hair loss.

254.   Increase the amount of folic acid in your diet. You can do this by adding vegetables and carrots to your diet. Folic acid is good for hair growth and the health of your hair. Besides eating better food in your diet you can also take a supplement that has folic acid in it.

255.   To help stave off hair loss be cautious with the types of chemicals and treatments you put on it. Many dyes have chemicals in them that are not good for your hair. Trust your hair to a licensed beautician, and you may be able to prevent some hair loss before it starts.

256.   Do everything you can to reduce the stress in your life. Stress can cause and also exacerbate hair loss. It is important to practice taking deep breaths to help yourself calm down and to find relaxing activities, such as reading, that you enjoy doing. If you can minimize the amount of stress in your life, you should see improvements in the quality of your hair.

257.   Consider having a hair transplant to correct your hair loss. This procedure is performed by a specialist, usually on men who are older than 35. Hair follicles from the back of the head are surgically removed and implanted in the bald areas. Although it is costly, hair transplants provide a

permanent natural looking solution to this vexing problem.

258.   Keep eating a lot of protein to slow down loss of hair. Many foods such as eggs, fish, poultry, nuts and beans supply much needed protein to your body. This gives your hair keratin, which is vital for growth. Keratin will help to strengthen your hair, and reduce future hair loss.

259.   In order to prevent your hair from falling out, you want to consider avoiding hair relaxers. The chemicals in these products are known to make hair fragile and fall out. Also, avoid using rollers in your hair. They grab onto hair too tightly and could cause it to fall out.

260.   For men that suffer excessive hair loss, liquid saw palmetto is a good non-prescription treatment to try. DHT is a male hormone thought to cause loss of hair; DHT growth is decreased by the natural extract found in saw palmetto. To use this natural method, extract juices from the fruit and apply it to your hair.

261.   It is vital to instill quality nutrients into your diet on a daily basis. With each of your meals during the day, make sure that you get a healthy dose of vegetables. Vegetables such as carrots will give your

hair the minerals it needs to function properly and maintain strength.

262.   In order to prevent your scalp from becoming dry when you're using a minoxidil product like Rogaine, make sure that you're using ample conditioner when you wash your hair. You need to keep your scalp moisturized. Having an excessively dry scalp may counteract the effectiveness of a product you're taking or using.

263.   There are two FDA-approved medications, Minoxidil and Finasteride, for treating inherited hair loss (androgenic alopecia).You can get Minoxidil (Rogaine) without a prescription. It is to sprayed or rubbed into the scalp twice daily. A prescription is needed for Finasteride (Propecia). Finasteride is not approved for women. It comes in pills to be taken once a day.

264.   If you have lost your hair and a wig isn't really your style, look into different types of hats and other head wear that you can use to make yourself feel better. It doesn't have to be a baseball cap or a Sinatra-like fedora. You can look into getting a turban or a scarf or some other type of head dress.

265.   Carbohydrate-rich food not only leads to weight gain in most people, it can also lead to hair loss in

many, so try to cut back on the carbohydrates if you want to keep more of your hair. Carbohydrates get converted by the body into sugar, and higher blood sugar can result in quicker hair loss.

266.   In order to help prevent hair loss, make sure you are getting enough protein in your diet. To keep your hair as healthy as possible, try to eat plenty of protein-rich foods as often as you can. Some good sources of foods rich in protein include eggs, seafood, bean sprouts, almonds, and fish.

267.   See your doctor. Before resigning yourself to thinning hair, consult with your primary care physician. There are numerous conditions from hypothyroidism to vitamin deficiencies that could be the cause of your hair loss. If the hair loss is due to an underlying condition, treating the condition is often enough to restore hair growth.

268.   When people experience hair loss, one of the most common culprits is using hair dryers. Too much hair drying at high temperatures can damage the hair structure, resulting in excessive hair loss. Some remedies are to blow dry the hair less often and towel or air dry instead.

269.   To control your risk of losing your hair, lower your risk of diabetes. Diabetes, like many diseases,

is a fairly common non-genetic reason for hair loss. Cut the amount of sugar in your diet, watch your weight, and make sure that if you do have diabetes, you control it well. These actions will all help prevent diabetes-related hair loss.

270.   Use baby shampoo to wash your hair. This is gentle on your hair and doesn't have many chemicals that can cause harm to your hair. You should make sure you don't shampoo your hair more than once a day. You also should be gentle with your hair when you wash it.

271.   Try using emu oil for your scalp and hair. Rub the oil on your scalp and through your hair before you go to bed.

272.   If you like to pull your hair back into a tight pony tail or other similar styles, then you could be causing your hair to thin. Having your hair tight like that causes the hair to grow closer to the surface than normal. If they are too close to the scalp surface, they may lose their hold and fall out.

273.   It is possible that chemicals can lead to hair loss. If you use chemicals on your hair, it is best to let a licensed beautician do it. They are able to properly perform chemical treatments to your hair. Also, if

you color your hair, do it no more than every 6 to 8 weeks.

274.   One of the things that you will want to do is limit dandruff, especially in the fall and winter. Dandruff may damage the texture and strength of your hair and can lead to excess dryness of your scalp. Purchase a shampoo that eliminates the cause of dandruff in a gentle way. You do not want to use a product that irritates your scalp either.

275.   Are you losing more and more hair each day? Are you fearing this hair loss will evolve into bald spots in the near future? One thing you can do to cut back on hair loss is the be more gentle with your hair when it is wet. Refrain from brushing or combing your hair roughly while it is wet. When wet hair roots are very weak and are prone to breakage.

276.   Help prevent hair loss by watching what you eat. Hair is essentially protein and needs to be fed protein to grow and thrive, however, watch the type of proteins you feed your body. Proteins that are high in fat, like steaks, tend to increase testosterone levels and that has been proven to cause hair loss. Opt for lean proteins like fish, beans and chicken for healthy hair.

277.   Carbohydrate-rich food not only leads to weight gain in most people, it can also lead to hair loss in many, so try to cut back on the carbohydrates if you want to keep more of your hair. Carbohydrates get converted by the body into sugar, and higher blood sugar can result in quicker hair loss.

278.   Most people think that hereditary hair loss is about hair falling out. Actually, it's about more hair not growing back to replace shed hair. Genetic hair loss can be caused by gender (men suffer more than women) age and hormones (testosterone). Unfortunately, men do suffer the most.

279.   Vitamin B deficiency not only helps increase hair loss, but it can also cause premature graying of the hair. Without the proper amounts of vitamin B, your scalp becomes oily, full of dandruff, and begins to bald. Make sure you have enough Vitamin B by eating vegetables, grains, beans, and more.

280.   If you can afford it, consider a hair transplant for your hair loss problem. Individual grafts of single strands of hair, or a Micrograft Hair Restoration Transplant, have proven successful in many patients. This is probably the closest simulation to having your own hair. Get full information from the transplant specialist before you go this route.

281.   To increase the health of your hair and possibly prevent hair loss, increase circulation to your scalp. You can do this by doing headstands, by giving yourself gentle scalp massages, by exercising, by breathing deeply or by improving your circulation in general. Better circulation to your scalp means more nutrients to your hair, and that means that you're more likely to avoid hair problems.

282.   Use baby shampoo to wash your hair. This is gentle on your hair and doesn't have many chemicals that can cause harm to your hair. You should make sure you don't shampoo your hair more than once a day. You also should be gentle with your hair when you wash it.

283.   To help treat hair loss related to a skin problem, consider including more essential fatty acids in your diet. In scientific studies, increased intake of omega-3 fatty acids and omega-6 fatty acids has sometimes shown improvement in hair loss related to a skin condition. Omega-3 foods include flax seeds, walnuts and salmon, and omega-6 foods include egg yolks and cooking oils. Keep the two types of fatty acids in proper balance for optimal results.

284.   You should not use just any shampoo for your hair. You have to be careful which products you use

on your hair. A good example is using a 3 in 1 shampoo, with a conditioner and body wash included. This could damage your hair, which could lead to it falling out prematurely.

285.   Use satin or silk pillowcases. Many people believe by using this material to sleep on can prevent hair loss. Using cotton or flannel pillowcases can cause your hair to pull. A satin or silk pillowcase will let your hair slide around and won't pull on your hair, causing hair loss.

286.   If you are having sudden hair loss that is unexplained, think about the stress you are dealing with in your life. Stress at home or at work is a common cause of hair loss, but you should be able to regrow your hair once you get stress under control.

287.   A helpful strategy to diminish or avoid hair loss is to adopt better hair care habits. Avoid excessive dyeing and harsh chemical treatment to your hair. Refrain or limit the amount of heat applied to your hair through the use of blow dryers, curling irons, straighteners, etc. All of the above cause breakage of the hair shaft and can result in hair loss also.

288.   Avoid brushing your hair when it's wet since that is the time it is most vulnerable. Brushing your

hair when it is wet causes more pull on your individual hair follicles causing a lot of your hair to be pulled out, even though they are healthy. The best policy is to just let your hair dry naturally when you can (except winter months or during cold weather).

289.   One of the best ways to limit hair loss is to reduce the amount of stress in your life. If you are at a job that puts you under a lot of pressure, make sure to practice stress relieving exercises during the day. This will make you feel better and help hair loss.

290.   For people that are suffering from hair loss and braid their hair frequently, you may want to consider giving your hair a rest. Having hair pulled back tightly, such as in braids or even a ponytail, can cause it to fall out. Try to wear your hair down as much as you can.

291.   Try using Rogaine or another solution that contains minoxidil to help prevent hair loss. This is a topical solution that must be applied to the scalp twice a day, and it can be used by both men and women. Many people notice that after several months of use, their hair loss ceases. Some even experience a regrowth of hair.

292.   Make sure to avoid shampoo products that
contain a lot of chemicals. These types of shampoos
not only dry your hair out but lead to split ends and
a damaged scalp. The next time you go to the drug
store, purchase a shampoo that is made up of
natural ingredients.

293.   If you are taking a bath or shower, try to stick to
lukewarm or cold water to wash your hair. Hot
water can strip all the oils from your skin, which can
yield the dryness and breakable hair. Only wash
with warm water if you desire to have a healthy
head of hair.

294.   The more you learn about different ways to
control hair loss and to boost growth, the more
you'll know about the side effects of the active
ingredients. Once you have completed your
research you may decide on a more expensive, yet
more effective option.

295.   Calcium is a great supplement to receive if
you're looking to strengthen your hair to prevent
further loss. Calcium is essential in creating and
strengthening bones, nails, and even the substance
hair is made out of, keratin. Make sure you're
including some calcium-rich foods or a calcium
supplement in your diet.

296. Volume-boosting shampoo can be your best friend if you're trying to give your head of hair a healthy boost. Some hair loss is fixed via cosmetic solutions, and working with a volume-boosting shampoo can be a fantastic way to make your head of hair look full, rich and illustrious even if it isn't.

297. Using apple cider vinegar on your hair can prevent hair loss. Its natural ingredients help to keep hair healthy and in place. To use it properly, heat up the apple cider vinegar slightly. Then, pour a little on your hair and wrap it in a towel. Let it sit for an hour and then wash it out.

298. It is best to use an all natural shampoo that is composed of herbal extracts. These shampoos do not clog hair follicles, and they actually increase hair retention as well as still maintaining manageability. These herbal shampoos cleanse hair the all natural way, and protect your hair rather than harm it.

299. What each individual needs for their nutrition depends on many factors including metabolism, age, diet, genetics, body size, and more. It is advised that you seek advice from a medical professional as to what vitamin supplements you might need to take in order to help you prevent or stop hair loss.

300. Try to reduce your level of stress on your body if you want to slow down your hair loss. When your body is under stress, your body channels energy into repairing the body instead of growing hair. So the rate of your hair growth slows, causing your hair to thin. Try to treat your body with more care and do not exert yourself. You might see an improvement in your hair growth.

301. Hormonal imbalance has been proven to be one of the main causes of hair loss. This is true in women as well. Pregnant women or women who have gone on and off birth control run a risk of hair loss, but this hair loss is usually temporary. Still, be aware of these concerns.

302. To prevent hair loss through nutrient deficiency, make sure to get enough of the amino acid lysine. Lysine deficiency has been linked to hair loss problems, while increased lysine intake has been linked to increased hair growth rate and decreased shedding of hair. Lysine is available in supplements, but is also found in foods, such as yogurt, cheese, beets and mangos.

303. Calcium is going to play a big role in whether you suffer from hair loss. Low levels of calcium in your diet could lead to weak hair follicles and hair roots which will cause your hair to begin to fall out.

Increase the amount of calcium in your diet to prevent the hair from falling out.

304.   To prevent hair damage that can lead to hair loss or thinning, don't use sulfates, formaldehyde or sodium chloride on your hair. These chemicals can sometimes be found in hair products like shampoo or styling products, and they're known to cause damage to the hair, which increases the rate of hair shedding and breakage.

305.   Massage your scalp. This helps with preventing hair loss and helps hair grow back. Massaging your scalp will help the blood and nutrients circulate in your scalp. Just rub your head with your fingers in a slow circular motion. When it gets warm and tingly it means the blood is flowing.

306.   To help prevent hair loss make sure to let your hair be loose and not confined as often as possible. Having your hair tied in elastics or tightly snug under a ball cap has been suggested as a cause for premature hair loss. As such avoid your hair being tightly confined.

307.   A healthy diet is not only good for your body, but it is also good for your hair. Eating healthy foods ensures that your hair gets all of the vitamins and minerals that it needs. Often the body to shows

poor health through the hair follicles and fingernails before it is shown in other parts of the body.

308.   Avoid stress at all costs if you don't want to lose your hair. Stress is one of the biggest causes of hair loss, and if you do not know how to control it, you will continue to suffer from hair loss. Learn to deal with your stress.

309.   Staying out in the sun too long can have a drying effect on your hair, which can eventually lead to balding. Make sure to limit your sun exposure, especially during the spring and summer. This will not only keep you safe, but will allow your hair to stay manageable and retain moisture.

310.   Natural herbal supplements to grow back your hair are the way to go for people who want to avoid the side effects associated with traditional medications. Some supplements will obviously work better than others, so you will need to test each one out individually to see what works best for you.

311.   A great way you can work to re-grow hair, and also prevent hair loss, is to massage your scalp regularly. Massage your scalp with oil to augment the effects of the massage on your hair follicles.

312.   Apply gentle massage techniques on the scalp to help promote healthier roots and hair growth. Be careful not to pull or tug at your hair in the process as this can pull out hair and cause breakage at the hair root. To ensure you don't pull your hair in the process, apply a conditioner before massaging to lubricate the scalp and rinse thoroughly when finished.

313.   Too much alcohol consumption can cause hair loss. A few drinks a week will not have an effect on your hair, but alcoholism does. If you are an alcoholic, there are many reasons to get help that is more important than hair loss. Talk to your physician and join Alcoholics Anonymous if you are battling an alcohol addiction.

314.   In order to mitigate hair loss or see a substantial decrease in hair loss you need to eat a healthier diet. This means you should eat more fruits, vegetables, beans, and non-fatty meats like fish and poultry. Stay away from complex carbohydrates because they produce sugars that are harmful to your body's balance.

315.   If you are suffering from hair loss, have a blood test done to check your iron levels. Excessive hair loss can be caused by anemia. If an iron deficiency is detected, your doctor can prescribe an iron

supplement for you. If there are no other underlying causes, taking the supplement regularly will most likely cure your hair loss problem.

316.   More than half of all men go through one form or another of hair loss after their mid twenties. DHT is a chemical that can destroy your hair, and you must take precautions to lessen your risk of losing your hair.

317.   Maintain a healthy diet. When your diet does not contain the right amount of nutrients your hair suffers. For a healthy head of hair, make sure you are consuming plenty of Vitamin A, C, and Omega-3 fatty acids. Vitamin A can be found in foods such as pumpkin, carrots and mango while Vitamin C can be found in most citrus fruits. You can get Omega-3 fatty acids in fish, nuts, flax seeds and olive oil.

318.   A surprising culprit of hair loss can sometimes be hormones. A hormonal imbalance, perhaps caused by birth control, can create hair loss. A temporary hormone imbalance may also be caused by hormone replacement treatment. Checking your hormone levels and monitoring them over time is an important step in identifying the causes of excessive hair loss.

319.   Try to avoid any types of toxins or pollutants if you want to improve hair quality. Harmful substances that find their way inside your body make you less healthy, and as your body struggles to stay healthy, this can have an adverse affect on your hair and contribute to its loss. Avoid breathing in toxic air and always wear plastic gloves when handling strong chemicals so they don't absorb into your skin.

320.   Keep your hair trimmed. By doing this you are taking dead ends off of your hair and it can grow longer and healthier. Dead ends can prevent your hair from growing any more and can make your hair weak and brittle. This can lead to hair loss in the future.

321.   To prevent hair damage that can lead to hair loss or thinning, don't use sulfates, formaldehyde or sodium chloride on your hair. These chemicals can sometimes be found in hair products like shampoo or styling products, and they're known to cause damage to the hair, which increases the rate of hair shedding and breakage.

322.   To get the best results from a wig, purchase one before you've lost all your hair. This will allow you to get a wig that matches your natural hair color exactly. This will also take some of the stress out of

hair loss. No matter what, you'll know you have a high quality wig you can wear at any time.